"What do you do if y[...] e insanely on fire with a vicious [...] take the chemo journey with[...] cause you are young, a wife and [...] hopes to live for other stories, you have no choice. You take the journey. And if you are a poet, you 'walk this poisonous way' hoping, praying, negotiating, and writing all the while. In this collection Katy moves through the halls of medicine and the corridors of pain to find she is only a 'tiny speck of glory, barely sparking,' but one carried in the arms of Jesus. Out of the crucible of cancer comes this rare collection of poems sure to be a comfort to any who have cussed, fought, and cried their way through an unwanted diagnosis or any of the heartaches and griefs common to humankind."

Margie Haack, author of *The Exact Place* and codirector of Ransom Fellowship

"Here is a writer who is as brilliant as she is brave; she brings us face-to-face with aches and joys that are so potent, they grip our hearts and refuse to let us run away from them. It is shocking how deeply personal yet widely relatable this body of work is. All in all, this is a very necessary book."

Moyosola Olowokure, artist and performance poet

"Writing from within the very heart of pain, exhaustion, and a search for meaning, Katy Bowser Hutson lays open her questioning heart in a way that a reader will want to join her in negotiating with God for survival and relief. This is profitable reading for those of us who want to do business with the God of salvation and healing."

Luci Shaw, poet and author of *The Generosity*

"Katy Bowser Hutson's poems and short essays are bodily and frank. Also, they are infused with light and hope that never feels sentimental. Into the valley of the shadow of death Katy speaks words of life. She is a gift, and these poems are a gift."

Jonathan Rogers, host of *The Habit Podcast* and The Habit Membership for Writers

"In this extraordinary book of poems, Katy Bowser Hutson names, knows, and faces the fear of cancer and all it contrives to take away. On each page, she steps through the unknowing, now resting, now fighting, always finding in language not just the death and darkness that follow from the fall, but also the grace that rises each day to meet it. 'I know the fall, and the overcome,' she writes. 'Running down fear with beauty,' she gives us a schooling in both. This book is a scarred gift, an unsentimental balm for the wounded, an illumination for us all."

Abram Van Engen, chair of the English department at Washington University and cohost of the *Poetry for All* podcast

"Both beautiful and harrowing, Katy Bowser Hutson's book takes readers on a journey into 'the depths.' In Hutson's case, they're the hellish depths of cancer, where senseless things are made sense of through the language of poetry—even if only partially—in order to discover a God who has not abandoned her to the depths but rather, in love, abided with her in them. This book is a gift to all who suffer and to those who keep watch with the sufferers."

W. David O. Taylor, associate professor of theology and culture at Fuller Theological Seminary and author of *Open and Unafraid*

"Katy's poetic reflections are unflinchingly honest—and stubborn in hope too. Whether you've received a cancer diagnosis or love someone who has, this book will help you feel less alone. These gentle invitations are full of quiet strength and will leave you with the profound truth that God's tender comfort is near, even in the most heart-wrenching moments of being human."

Kayla Craig, author of *Every Season Sacred* and *To Light Their Way*

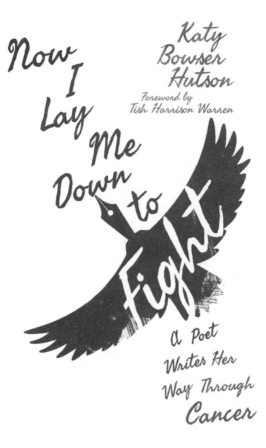

Now I Lay Me Down to

Fight

Katy
Bowser
Hutson

Foreword by
Tish Harrison Warren

A Poet
Writes Her
Way Through
Cancer

An imprint of InterVarsity Press
Downers Grove, Illinois

InterVarsity Press
P.O. Box 1400 | Downers Grove, IL 60515-1426
ivpress.com | email@ivpress.com

Cover design: David Fassett
Interior design: Daniel van Loon
Cover images: © CHRISTOPH BURGSTEDT / SCIENCE PHOTO LIBRARY / Getty Images, © CSA Images / Getty Images

ISBN 978-1-5140-0799-0 (print) | ISBN 978-1-5140-0800-3 (digital)

Printed in the United States of America ♾

Library of Congress Cataloging-in-Publication Data
Names: Hutson, Katherine J., 1977- author.
Title: Now I lay me down to fight : a poet writes her way through cancer / Katy Bowser Hutson.
Description: Downers Grove, IL : IVP, [2023]
Identifiers: LCCN 2023021623 (print) | LCCN 2023021624 (ebook) | ISBN 9781514007990 (paperback) | ISBN 9781514008003 (ebook)
Subjects: LCSH: Breast–Cancer–Poetry. | Hutson, Katherine J., 1977–Health. | Breast–Cancer– Patients–Biography. | Christian biography–United States. | LCGFT: Autobiographical poetry.
Classification: LCC PS3608.U873 N69 2023 (print) | LCC PS3608.U873 (ebook) | DDC 811/.6 [B]–dc23/eng/20230703
LC record available at https://lccn.loc.gov/2023021623
LC ebook record available at https://lccn.loc.gov/2023021624

29 28 27 26 25 24 23 | 12 11 10 9 8 7 6 5 4 3 2 1

In loving memory of my dear friend

LESLIE BUSTARD

CONTENTS

FOREWORD

Tish Harrison Warren

*W*hat would you do if you found out you may die soon? My friend Katy turned to what she had spent her life doing: shaping words, asking questions, trusting God and doubting him and trusting again, and eking out beauty from the ashes.

When facing the darkness of our mortality and fragility, we need theologians, but we also—and more so—need poets. We need those who help us to notice any hint of light in the darkness. We need faithful men and women who with pen in hand act as spelunkers, plunging into the dark caves of human experience, exploring what we would rather avoid, and telling us what they found there.

The fact is that any of us may die soon. And very likely, all of us, even if we make it several more decades, will still feel that life is short and that it's all too soon to go. This collection will serve as a boon and a guide not only to those facing cancer but to all of us who face our own dark nights—our own calls to lay down and fight.

As Katy once wrote in her lovely review of one of my books, I am not an unbiased reviewer or judge of this work. How could I be? Katy is one of my dear friends. I'm even mentioned in one of these poems. Still, what strikes me about these verses is how much of my friend's spirit made it into them. Reading these poems will feel like sitting down with a friend even for people who have never met Katy—sitting with a friend to hear about the kind of wisdom that can only be hard won, both in the tears and in the surprising moments of grace and joy.

My husband and I cried when we found out that our friend Katy had a particularly aggressive and deadly form of cancer. We wept for her and for her husband and children, and the heartbreaking and uncertain journey ahead. What we could not see in that moment of tears was how our friend would find mercy in a chemo clinic and how she would live to tell the rest of us about it. We could not see how Jesus was waiting for our friend and her family in places that no one would ever choose to go.

The poems in *Now I Lay Me Down to Fight* are luminous, honest, heartbreaking, and, at moments, even funny. They are at once defiant yet surrendered, buoyant yet profound, faithful yet never trite. To read them is to encounter a beautiful and brave soul who invites us into her vulnerability, illness, and mortality through images and stories, as human as they are hopeful. I cried reading these verses—no surprise given the subject and my love for the poet. What did surprise me was how much I smiled as well. Katy Hutson has descended into the darkness of cancer and there wrought beauty, goodness, wisdom, and even abundance.

PREFACE

The Week Before Cancer

One of the worst days of my life followed one of the best weeks. I'd just completed a week at the Martha's Vineyard Institute of Creative Writing, courtesy of a scholarship from the Sustainable Arts Foundation for artists with young children. After a long stretch of homeschooling young children, writing music, and holding down the fort while my husband was on the road playing music, this week was an utter godsend: a week to rest, write, learn, and make plans for my next creative steps when I returned home. To drag out the trope, little did I know . . .

That evening, as I got ready for bed at a friend's house in Boston, I saw warning signs on my body: my breast was hot, swollen, puckered. Within a week I was in chemotherapy for a rare, aggressive cancer called inflammatory breast cancer.

I felt an immediate awareness that there was no accident in the timing. The week of honing my writing skills had given me tools in my arsenal for this battle.

In his book *The Body Keeps the Score*, psychiatrist Bessel van der Kolk notes that trauma is preverbal. There is a magic, a medicine to putting words to terrible things. I wrote through all of it: to face fear, to say it out loud, to pray, to fling it all away from me. I wrote most of the poems during cancer treatment. The essays, as well as one poem, are written with the benefit of hindsight, five years later. My hope is that my writings cross paths with someone who could use these words. Every cancer story is different. Maybe there are moments in here that resonate, that help. I hope so.

BEGINNING

*M*ake no mistake: without treatment, this is fatal." In order to save my life, my oncologist made it quite clear that without her help, this was how I would die. There was no optimistic assurance that I was going to live. That's one thing I had that most people don't have: knowledge of how I would die. Maybe.

Cancer is a memento mori. I've had a sturdy stare down with death, which changed me. To the best of my knowledge, I don't have cancer now. But if you've had cancer, you know you're never free of it. Not really. I often tell people that I feel like Frodo Baggins after he's been wounded by a wraith— the hurt will always be with me. Or maybe like the apostle Paul, with the thorn in his flesh (2 Corinthians 12:7). That feels a bit holier. There was a point, after all, when a person literally could put their finger in the wound in my side. Although it wasn't advisable.

Five years down the road, I still have lots of souvenirs from treatment. My torso is a battlefield of scars. I can't quite feel the tips of my toes, a parting shot from chemo. The skin on my chest is still fused to my breastbone in places. The surgeon had to sever nerves in order to remove lymph nodes under my arm, so my son likes to run his finger down the back of my arm where I can't quite feel to figure out where the feeling starts and give me the heebie-jeebies. And I just get tired easily.

I wrote these thoughts for me, to survive. To fling out the fear and sadness onto a page where I could look at them and have more control and understanding. Where I could admit them and yell them and pray them. I hope they help you, too. I wouldn't presume to know the ways cancer wounds others, any more than I'd presume to know how to treat it. But sorrow shared is half sorrow, right? And joy shared is double joy. Strangely, joy can even thread itself through terrible things. I'll go as far as to say that some joys can only be known in sorrow.

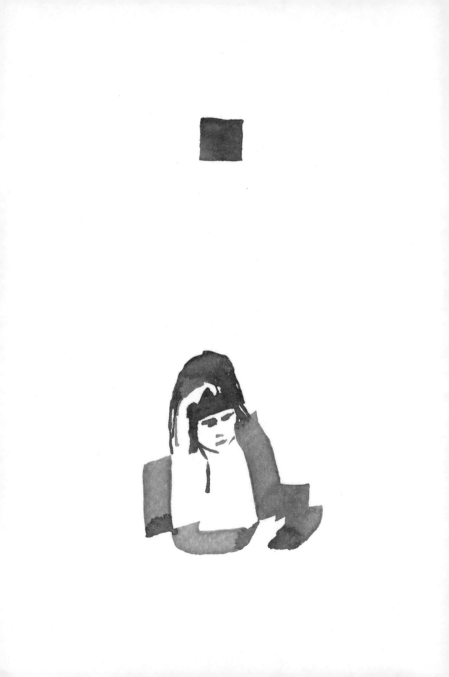

FUMBLE FINGERED

Written a few days before diagnosis

This world doesn't work well for us
God spins it just fine,
But we are fumble fingered.
The cells are broken deep down.

We fuss with fixing spaceships with chopsticks
And numb our nerves
With pixels and ethers.

PREPARATION

*Written the day before diagnosis, while
attending the Martha's Vineyard Institute
of Creative Writing*

I go home tomorrow, leave Martha's Vineyard
Where I sleep till I wake
Catbirds and mourning doves sing at 4:30 a.m.
Go sleep, go sleep
Here no heavy little blond hot water lies across my trunk,
Cheek to cheek
Just breathing my waking breath.
"Hey mama. I cuddle you."
Then the honey haired six year old stumbles in
Rubbing the sleep out, complaining it's bright
The fighting begins, jockeying for the cuddliest spot on
mama.
The three year old hits the six year old,
The six year old howls indignantly

Three chickens wait—two taffeta black sheened girls
Golden Little Miss Muffin who doesn't know she's
beautiful
I am their dealer, doling out oats and mealworms
My husband who sits with me by the fire out back at night:
He has the most words at the end of the day.

I've made habits these past five days
I wake, make coffee, drink it, dress
Walk my brain and body a mile to the bus
Past privileged sheep and high-born horses
Round the rocky curve where
Three centuries or so of ghosts
Whose headstones are wind and rain worn
Eroding like salty shores
Easily erased from current memory
I've been etching something this week, more ephemeral
Than the final tributes to Athea, Isadora, Adelaide and all
those Mayhews.
I am wrangling words into a daisychain
To garland my daughter's brain
To whisper in her perfect ear
When she's leaning her bony shoulder in my ribs
Cheek on my chest
"Mama, tell me about Jack and Eliza"
I'll unzip my suitcase and bring her home a seashell and a
story.

MEETING MY ONCOLOGIST

Waiting waiting in the room of a doctor
The very good recommended doctor
As cancer is in my body
I wait for her, my general, to tell me the lay of
The battlefield.
Hello, so thankful to meet you:
Can you save my life?
If ever a first impression felt important.
All of the previous stories we both have.
Do you know?
How many battles waging?
How many fronts lost?
Can we rally?
Can we retaliate?
Can we win the day?
Do I live?
This beige room has no clues.

I looked her up
She digs deep into new questions.
She has children.
She looks kind.

Words, I know.
I know people.
Not cells much.
Not treasonous cells.
Not heroic cells.
But I know the fall, and the overcome.
A low timpani roll rising to crescendo.
We are past the cymbals and trumpets
In the long, certain denouement
Fraught with casualties
Foes getting in punches on the run.

EN ROUTE TO CANAAN/JERICHO

Cancer and its accompanying stats
Can lead a person into the foolish wrestling match
Of a negotiation with God.
If I beat the thirty-three percent odds of dying
in the next three years,
Can I stick around to finish teaching my children?
How about writing my book?
How about to travel with Kenny?
Can I forgo my "high chance of recurrence"
And be there when my community needs me to speak bravely
Or create sacrificially?
Or hold my daughter's hand?

Body, soul, listen up:
This is the same damned deal as before.
You've always had a death sentence.
You've always had the same odds.
You didn't know what they were,
But now someone has given you some vague lottery ticket
pulled from a front car tire,
Pulpy and pitted.
But, for all you know,
you could still get hit by a drunk driver,
Struck by lightning
Fall dead of an aneurysm

Your cells could still go singingly along in symphony
til one hundred
and ten
Blissfully barely blinking through benign decades,
Blessedly bearing burdens you have enough for at every turn.
Which will embolden your prose,
Which will sharpen your sight,
Which will add pique to your poems,
Which will add intensity to your touch,
Kindness, forthrightness to your mouth,
Empathy to your eyes?
Which will draw love out of you?

Apparently: this poisonous path.
Bare me, bear me, Lord.
Pie Jesu, parry with this pilgrim
I hereby give up this particular thumb-wrestle
I am laid on my back
It was never any different since you took me in hand:
Every hair on my head, every hair broken off.
I have always malfunctioned in a malignant mire
And you have always raised me, wiped me, breathed in me,
Strapped me on the back of a donkey and taken me to the
Four Seasons
With medical miracle makers for my wounds.
You stuffed a million bucks in my pocket
And said you'd come back for me in a bit:
Order the room service.

CHEMOTHERAPY

I started chemotherapy immediately after diagnosis. Inflammatory breast cancer multiplies over days—we were racing the clock. My oncologist was a force of nature. I imagined that cancer cells heard her red stiletto heels clicking toward my room and trembled. She looked at my diagnosis on her screen, went to the door, and yelled down the hall for a nurse. She instructed the nurse to read the lab the riot act: We need my labs *yesterday*. We need to get chemo in my body *now*.

The next day, I had a port inserted to deliver my infusions. As I was being prepped for anesthesia, they told me that the device would go on the right side of my clavicle, and I felt a wave of sadness roll over me. My weaned boy still cuddled and fell asleep on my right side, and I feared we would lose that deep comfort which we would both need, more than ever. (I can't write this without crying.) Feeling desperate and audacious—a feeling I quickly grew into—I asked, hardly able to speak, if the port could go on my left side. The nurse's eyebrows raised, and she went to investigate. Apparently, she learned, it could. (Lesson learned: Always ask. If they say no, ask why.) The next day, I started chemo. Tick, tick, tick.

Chemo was waves. Like one of those gravity-powered roller coasters. Up and down and up and down, every high a little lower, every low a little lower until all momentum is gone and you fall into bed. The wisdom I heard from women who'd gone before me was to let the chemo do its work. Trust the work that's happening in you, conserve your resources. Rest. Lay down.

CHEMO POEM #1

Let's try writing with music on.
Let's try writing during chemo.

Two weeks ago, I wrote by the ocean.
Ridiculous prima ballerina sunsets
laying their souls out
inches across ocean
Gloriously arched over backwards
Illumining footlight waves
Past the overpriced fish and chips
Salty air and malt vinegar
Ocean eternal
I wrote and wrote
easy words and seashores of time

Two weeks later, I write in chemo.
With Goldberg Variations infusing through my headphones
Running down fear with beauty
With Trastuzumab infusing through my body's tunnels
Like some Cossack mob
Conquering and burning over-populating cells run amok

I can't say I like this better
But I can't say it's worse for writing.
Pain works just fine
Fear close as a CT scan suits
My days were measured before
Everybody's always are
The curtain's just pulled back a bit.
I always needed a deadline to get anything done.

CANCER, POET

Cancer is an overgrowth, a kudzu:
Tangling and strangling legitimate life.

Chemo is a killing, a burning out:
Burning down to ashy carbon, indiscriminately.

But cancer, did you know that I am a poet?
My job is to cull through the chaos
with tweezers and magnifier.
I have wings
On shoulder blades and ankles
Just big enough for hovering me inches above the terrain,
Traversing without smothering my subject.
With pen and pocket and fingers and eyes
I cipher meaning
Siphoning liquid beauty that seeps from the edges
Into a tiny vial;
Taking pains with my pain: it fruits sweetly.

If in this year's ravaging I eke an ounce of beauty
It will outweigh all of your ashy remnant.
I can paste it on my footsoles
And stick me to the incinerated earth
Where I will wait for the rich loam
Tear soaked and fertile, to live.
That is what poets do, cancer.

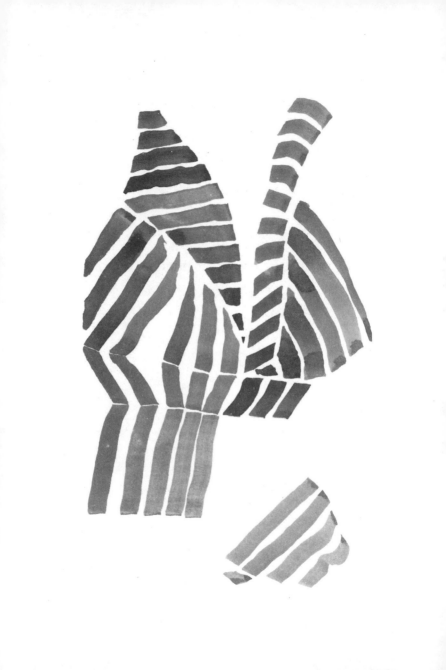

I WISH, I MISS, I THANK YOU

Today, I wish I had enough energy to play with my little boy.
But, today you have ordained that my guts reject food
And I will trust that you have done this on purpose,
That it is for my good.

Today, I wish I could be in a pumpkin patch with my daughter
She is playing with her cousins, and that is a good, good gift
I will praise you for it from my bed.
Your gifts are good

I miss my hair today,
I'm grieving the takeover of my breasts
But I do not need them, or I would have them.
I was never promised to make it
through this world without battle scars
But you have promised to carry me safely through,
heart safely tucked away in your own
Where no cancer, no doubt, no decay can get at it to harm it.

You never promised me that I would get to finish
all of my creative projects.
But you do let me make, and I apologize for when
I have been lazy
I thank you that you have indeed let me create, for good.

I thank you for my family, who are caring for my children,
our home—
My mom, who keeps washing my sheets and making my bed.
My dad, who is painting my kitchen and making it sweet
and lovely.
My husband, holding it all together, falling apart with me.
I thank you for this bed.

PREPOSITION

Eating from bed tonight
It's staying down.
I'm staying down.
The sun is down and I've been down all day.
All the drugs are in,
Keeping everything in.

Mom is putting the dishes away
Dad put a coat of paint on the cabinets
Kenny rode on a plane,
Played on a stage
And is riding on a bus.

I am in a bed.
The chemo is in me.
The cancer might be in me
But it might not.

The kids are coming home
My girl goes on a plane tomorrow
To be with cousins
We'll keep our boy home
And spoil him

Now the drugs are in
I'm down for the count
Feels like losing
But it's working
So I submit
I bow.

I will always have a shadow of a doubt,
A thorn in me,
A cloud around my heart
So I will need you, Jesus.
I have a bracelet around my wrist
Tish gave it to me yesterday, to pray
Lord Jesus Christ, Son of God, have mercy on me, a sinner
Around and around and around.

IMBALANCE/BALANCING

With thanks to the scientists at Genentech,
creators of Herceptin

Cancer and global warming:
Cut from the same cloth.
Things are a degree too cold, and some species dies
An inch too close to the sun, some spore proliferates.
A million reasons to be out of whack.
A wonder I ever made it this long without cancer
A wonder that I'm living on this side of the date
That provided a miracle molecule,
An estrogen receptor dismantler
My cancer is one hundred percent fatal without treatment
Fifteen years ago I could be one hundred percent gone
The world keeps spinning and I was dropped on precisely
this point in space and time, unbelievably micro-placed
If space goes up and time goes out:
It is a big dark mass
But
It has a tiny, bright, hopeful spot in the corner
And there I dance on the head of a pin
    through no fault of my own

Chemo is not pretty
Infections are not pretty
Losing breasts is not pretty
Radiation is not pretty
But a beating heart is pretty
A tumor that shies from Herceptin is breathtaking
A mind that can enjoy the massive miracle of my tiny
    toe-tip
tract of history
The beginning of a silver line drawn by modern medicine
Takes my breath away: it's a good view.

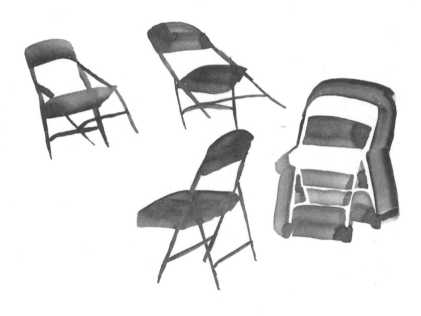

SLEEP AS WAR

I will not begrudge the bad days
For then are the vehicles valiant
Victorious in throes of carcinoma
Then the rank rotting reels
There the nuisance is nevered away

Now I lay me down to fight,
Rest in God with all his might.
I have no claim upon tomorrow,
Today is joy, and war and sorrow.
Fiercely now the battle's joined
In axillary node and groin
Meta, micro, in between
Trusting that which is not seen.

CHEMO POEM #2

The nurse in chemo infusion
Likes that I'm a poet
Because I can say
"I can still breathe,
　but it feels like my sternum has turned into a lead plate."
She compliments how descriptive I am.
It's the best I've got.

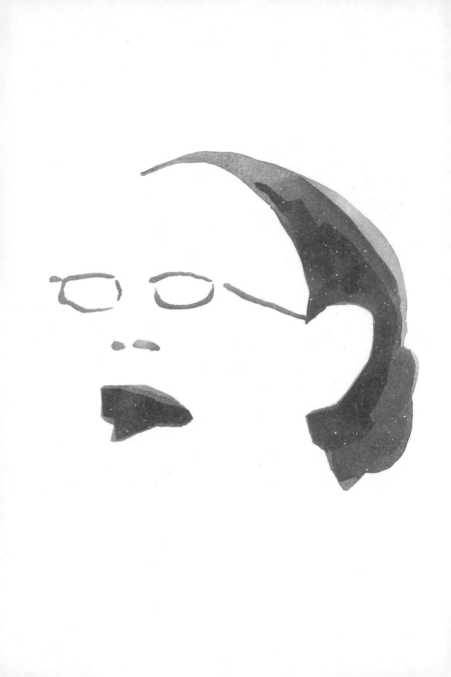

ROUND TWO CHEMO

Second verse,
Same as first.
Except worse.

I am in bedagainbedagainbedagain
Missing parties
And fresh air

My littles come and cuddle me
The blue-eyed hot water bottle
Climbs in next to me
For a sleepover with mama
Cold chubby feet
On my bed-warm thighs

Half a hamburger in three days
I just asked for fish sticks
They sounded crunchy, salty, greasy
But two bites in they are fishy
And I can't even think of s_____ without feeling sick.

Round two chemo
Second verse,
Same as first.
Except worse.
Taut and terse.

Cracked the window for some air
Cicadas crescendo, disappear
No birds—taking a union break
While the bugs fill in during this August intermission

We're at the point where
I don't ask for my meds when I feel like them,
When I suspect they'd succour and assist.
Mom and Kenny just keep giving them to me on schedule
Because I do need them.
Keep me sleepy, settled, sedentary
Keep me safe and solid
Flow the fluids, food doesn't matter so much.

Del tells me to get up and use my legs.
Watch, son: let me wait on the chemo to curse the cancer
I will walk and hold you and plank my muscles into strength
And hug you with hard hugs
And kiss every pink inch of your face.
We will hike and creekwalk and read a million books
And help and write and listen to good stories and make music
And defy death.

UNCERTAINTY

The uncertainty of cancer in my body
It is just the flip side, isn't it
Of the mystery of the body we've proclaimed for years
Through ritual and habit,
Feasting and fasting

But uncertainty is just the same mystery, the same truth
Colored blue,
Blotted with fear instead of hope.

Uncertainty assumes a lack of control,
Control in malicious hands, in death's hands.
When said that boldly, though,
We see it's just unfounded fear.
It smacks of heresy.

SANGUINE

By the way, don't let me fool you.
I run on the half glass full side,
But I have fears.
I just face them, and answer them, and keep going.
They take time, and I don't know how much time I have.
I have things I'd rather do.
I don't think it's denial, but I do say that a lot,
And maybe I protest too much.
But they peek out from the corners of my mind
From the closets
They whisper
Sometimes just the facts
Dry and concrete
Sometimes more sinister,
More whispy and mysterious
I deal better in that realm,
In the nethers and ante-spaces
The fears are there. I just don't have time to feed them.
I don't know if I have time, actually—
Look, there's another fact/fear.
They're all woven through.
But they'll have to come along for the ride and hang on—
I have things to do.

TRAINING

I am as strong as my stomach
Gurgling and grasping but never really gathering
On the bathroom floor
The sun still shying up pre-dawn
It's a Thursday
Sitting in the bathroom floor,
Potty-training Del
Enduring chemo stomach
Hoping I don't need to push him off the potty
You are all my strength and glory

BLESS YOUR HEART

That was thoughtful, chemo,
to pass on symptoms til after
the children were in bed.
The glands in my neck, shoulders, upper back,
Growling like gremlins
Fighting while the children weren't watching
I tried to take a one-handed picture of
    my boy and my brother;
My hand shook beyond settling.
But that was as bad as it got.

ERASER

Losing my hair:
No big deal, really.
Eyelashes, on the other hand, scared me.
The shadows, the depth of my face
Erased.
Blanking me out

Blankety-blank cancer
Already attempting to flatten me
Into a one dimensional character

I have other stories to tell
I have things to do
I'm a beauty bearer
Where you, cancer, copy furiously,
I fumblingly create.
You cannot uncreate me.

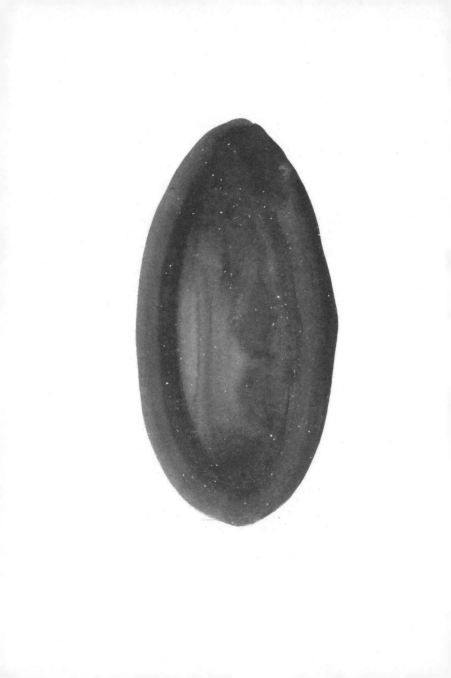

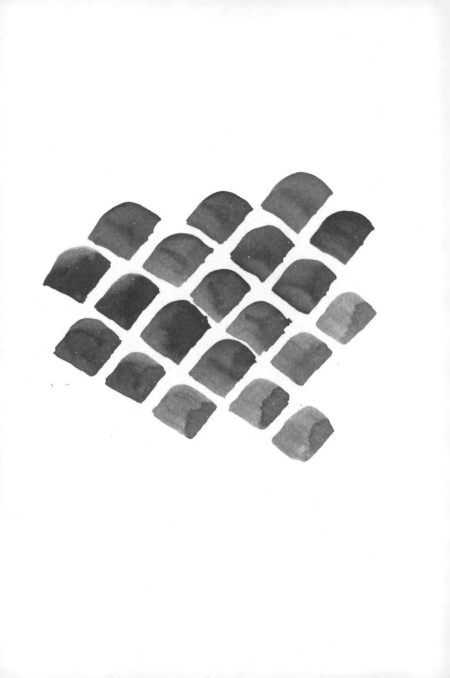

TREATMENT IS A GAUNTLET

Treatment is a gauntlet,
battering at each attempt.
To the victor goes the spoils:
The life you've been living,
That you never quite knew you wanted so badly.
Let them stick you, amputate parts of you,
Pump you with medicines and chemicals,
Let them explore you, help you.
You alone are the vision-keeper of what your life is.
You, and your Maker and your dear ones.

WASHCLOTH

I am a worn out washcloth
Wrung too tight
Till the fibers frayed
Not fit for the nice linens
Relegated to the rag bin
Twisted and left to dry stiff
Such that, once washed
I will never be square again

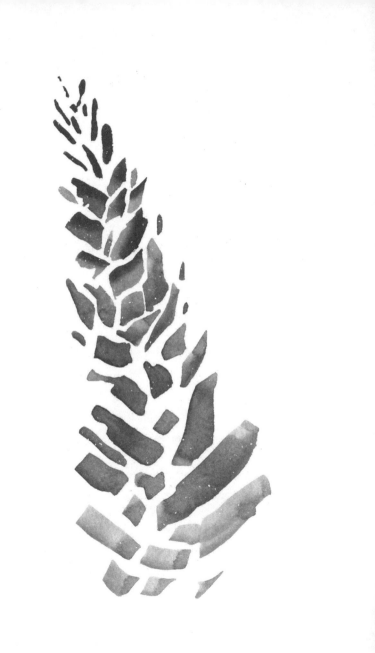

POTTY MOUTH

I euphemize to minimize
And keep my head above my gut
My gut, which decided that shit trumps poetry this morning.

All settled in with tea and notebook and book
Favorite nook, finally alone, out, by myself.
Rumbling and cramps, bastard bowels:
"Sorry, high-minded girl.
I've decided that mere merde will rule."
Vicious visceral reaction.
Indignity delivered by a thousand little humblings.

Body of death.
Muttering and murderous thoughts.
An apology from the sanitation department:
"Sorry, the sewer's out of order,
We need to close the library for the duration.
We apologize for any inconvenience."

Jerk body. Jerk GI.
Sigh.
God-made body.
Precious body.
Held hostage body.
Jerk cancer.
Jackass cancer.

Brutal mercenary chemo: do your thing.
But can you remember you're on my side?

We made a deal, but it's dangerous dealing with mobsters.
You hear what you want to hear.
You get my hair: I feel a little noble
 looking like I'm going to be burned at the stake.
You get my flora,
You get all my extra energy, at least half the time.
You get my guts.
 Can you choose your timing?
That was classless.
But mobsters don't deal in subtleties.
Well, shit.

METASTASIS

My cancer metastasized into my dream last night.
A white puppy with brown spots chased my chickens
And as I chased him off he scampered through the hedge,
Through an unlocked fence door and into the neighbor's yard.
I followed unwittingly through
harried but cheerful
I explained to the scrawny young couple next door
That their puppy had made an attempt on my chickens.
The young man looked put off and rolled his eyes
As he jumped into their swampy pool,
His wife diapered their scrawny baby.
Exasperated, I tried explaining:
their side gate had been unlocked,
The puppy (whom I had just returned)
Had tried to eat my hens.
No hard feelings, but—
"Fine," he said, "but if this all just a bit of drama . . ."
I felt my head start to sweat and pulled off my hat.
Running my hand over my shaved head.
He looked and his manner changed.

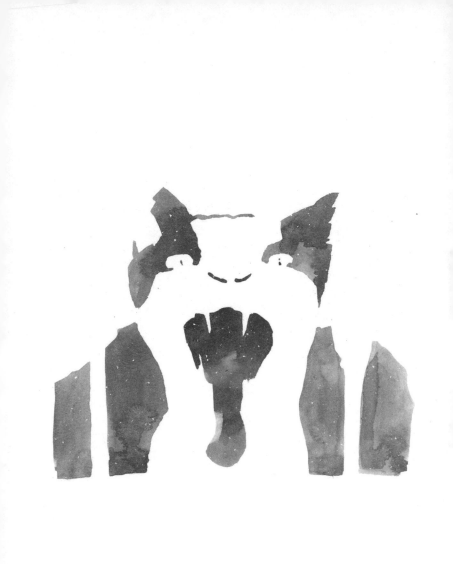

FRUSTRATION

I am frustrated, and need to clarify.
I feel frustrated, but I don't mean that.
I am making an accusation:
I have been frustrated, therefore I am in a state of frustration.
You have frustrated me,
You have allowed me to be frustrated.
One or the other, either way.
I had plans, I had hopes,
I rather figured they were in line with yours.
I was mistaken, maybe.
Maybe not. Is this your take on how we get there?
You can see ten days into the future, ten years.
I am not worried about one hundred or one thousand years,
I know you've got those.
But this cancer route:
It is frustrating.

The children are getting more self-sufficient,
I was getting more unscrambled, stronger, more resilient.
My dreams had become plans with steps, I had thrown out lessers
And was making steps on greaters.
Now I have a boot on my neck.
Are you making me tougher, making it so I make it through my work?
Survival training?
I'll take it if you tell me it is.
I'll take it if you don't.
I am tempted to add conditions and caveats,
But there's no setting up my sandcastles
on the shores of your citadels.

HMS *ONDANSETRON*

Another morning in bed
The window's cracked two inches,
Just begging a bird to sneak in.
The rain patters plat-plat outside
On the flat, shiny holly

When I sit still here
I imagine I could just hop up
I pretend I'm just lazing.
I think, "Maybe I'll just hop up and
Do some pushups
Or hop in the car and go on a quick errand
Or go for a walk."

But I forgot that I am shipwrecked
The carpet slips and tilts when I stand.
The floor leans.
I am on a raft, then:
Floating, floating, safe and dry.

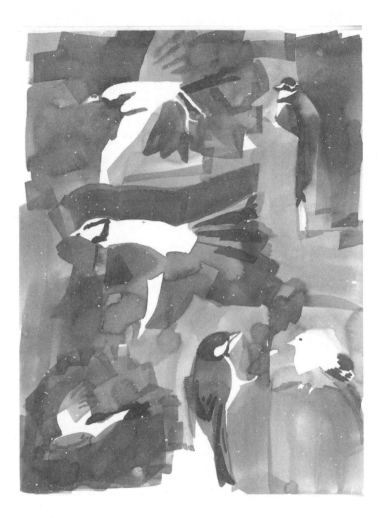

3

MASTECTOMY

*B*reasts are . . . tender. Women bless and curse them. They hurt our backs. They make it harder to exercise. They feed our babies in magical ways. They give us and our lovers pleasure. They draw attention, welcome or otherwise. And still, somehow, losing my breasts was the easiest part. Maybe because it was the most visible signifier that something proactive was happening.

From the moment I found out my breasts were occupied territory, I didn't think twice about losing them to save my life. I only had cancer in my right breast but asked the surgeon to please take both. Whatever it takes to never do this again. And while we were at it, I made it clear that I didn't have any interest in reconstruction—I've got other things I'd rather do with that time. (I know that's not true for everyone. Breasts are wonderful, of course. Except if they are, as the bumpers stickers and tank tops say, trying to kill you.)

Even though I bid my embattled breasts good riddance, I grieved their loss. My precious body, the body who carries me around this world, born from my mother and bearer of my two children. My body who has held my friends, dug gardens, written, sung. My God-made body who has done so many good and hard things. Part of her is gone. (One comfort in my marriage is that my husband is also an amputee: he lost an eye. It's nice that he understands.)

I forget all the time that I have a flat chest. I forget that other people notice, until someone reminds me. I was roller skating with my family recently when a fellow mom asked me if I was a survivor. I asked her how she knew, and she glanced at my flat chest with a raised eyebrow and smirk like, "Really?" We laughed. She was a survivor, too.

I don't feel any less female without breasts. Or ovaries, for that matter. Faced with the loss of some of my distinguishing female anatomy, I feel as though parts of my spiritual makeup as a woman became more pronounced during cancer. I bend in the face of difficulty with more grace, sometimes. I rise with more strength, sometimes. I've gone to war, and I am changed. My sternum feels like a breastplate now. I'm tired, but I am alive, and keenly aware that my days are gifts. When I forget, my body reminds me.

CONCERNING THE REMOVAL
OF MY BREASTS

It's time to take a good look at losing my breasts.
At least, sometime soon it is.
It never really seems like a good time,
But it is a fixed point on my lifeline before which
I will have breasts,
After which I will not.

I remember the first time I could tell others were aware
That I was wearing a bra
I was in Germany, I was eleven,
we were in a Gasthaus ordering dinner
And wearing a pink Land's End turtleneck
And it caught someone's eye
And I turned red from the neck up

Then it's a question of how to acknowledge them as an adult
A point of beauty, a delineation of my shape.
Finally, breasts, you fed my babies,
For twenty-seven months each.
You delivered some wizard-woven magic milk
That talked both ways: listening to my children's needs,
Changing the concoction accordingly.
I am so grateful, I am so proud, I am in wonder.

Just before the realization of cancer in my breasts,
I told my friend I'd been thinking about breasts,
how at this season it'd be nice to be able to just
Screw them off and put them on the shelf much of the time.
This is a season for doing, for creating, for working.
Breasts feel largely superfluous.
Not always, but largely.
They do not feel primary to my femininity,
To my humanity.

So, there it is! Off they will come.
Whether the second needs to go is debatable,
But I say let's make a clean breast of it.
Let's make it through scarred and brave and keeping what's
Worth keeping and by all means throw off what hinders.

BUS

"You deserve to be paid for what you've gone through."
This banner, a prophetic message to just me,
Just rolled by the window in a rainbow fade
On the side of a bus.
It was talking to me
Right?
Those geniuses, those liars, those prophets, those madmen.
Yeah, I do.
Deserve to be paid what:
There's the rub.

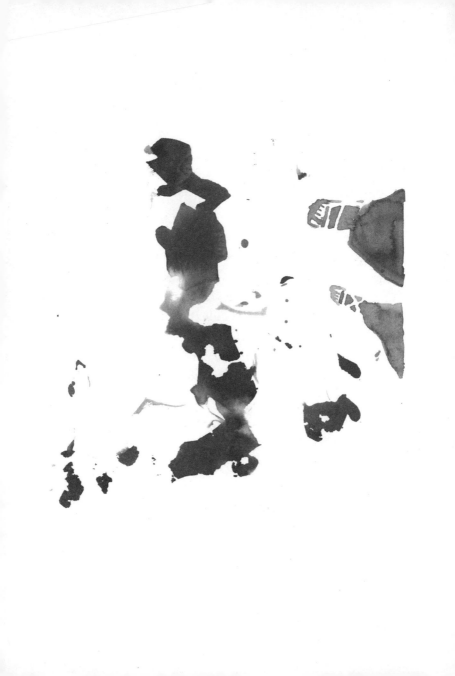

MASTECTOMY EVE

Do other people prepare their bodies for surgery?
For a naked, unconscious first impression?
I suspect 6–10 people whom I've never met will see my naked
body.
What can they know about me while I'm prone and inert?
My rings are off, but there's an indention there.
I trimmed my fingernails, striped from chemo.
My body has extra weight on it from weird eating and steroids.
I have scars on my breasts and clavicle from biopsies.

Do they make assumptions?
Of course they do.
I do.

Maybe I could write them a note on my stomach.

I wanted to wear my own socks
I brought unicorn socks—so they could see I have whimsy.
I brought hand-knit socks so they could see I am loved.
But I have to wear hospital socks with tire treads.
I hope my face has love lines on it,
I hope they see that I like my body and I'd like to keep it.

AFTER MASTECTOMY

I blipped into waking
A skipping record
Singing Holy, Holy, Holy

Pricks and sticks and snips and
Twinges and twitches and tenderness
I did nothing but sleep

My breasts are gone
They did their job
They were occupied territory so they had to go
Will I get them back when everything's all right again?

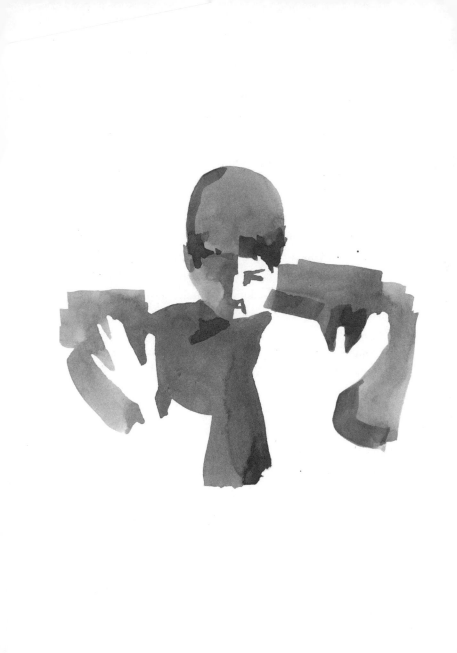

RUNNING ACROSS THE PAGE

I begin here. I start, I stumble, I stutter, I get some manner of
something that's not nothing out.
There's a new glove on my hand. It's stiff, my fingers snap back. It's
hard work. Is it healing work?
I stumble around, I get up again. Mentally stagger, physically push
forward, fingers faster than thinking. Catch up, head. Fingers are
incapacitated, held back but doing it anyway. Can you do it anyway?
Do it anyway. Just get it all out of your head. Just dump it, compost.
Dump it on the compost heap, let it get hot and simmer. Just move.
You don't have to have a plan. You just need to not let the stopping
stop you. You need to hold on to your hat and move forward in time
with a trail of trying in your wake.
Fragments falling off, folding in on yourself, falling out of yourself.
You don't even know what you mean, Katy.
Go faster. Don't let reason try to catch up.
You think you're so clever.
You think it takes a convent, you think it takes someone outside of
you.
But you stand Coram Deo and you must begin there—
Stop looking away and avert your eyes.
Raise your gaze just to lower it, glory-blind again.
You tiny speck of glory, barely sparking.

You mighty mankinder, kind of mankind, kind of kinder kid
Is this the best we've got?
Is this the best I've got?
No of course not obviously no. You are at the end of yourself and
have no genius to give
And you are being contrary and you think that you have to get it right
but Katy, you really have nothing right now. Not much. Stop and
shake it out. Don't medicate, don't judge, don't presume. Just run.
Run across the page. Fingers and buttons and clicking and clacking
and running across and down ropes on ropes of words all tangled and
tailend frayed made messy mope ropes muddled up muddled down.
Enough, never enough. But not intended to be, not made to be.
Never enough. So run into the enough and find out if it holds, if it's
strong enough, enough enough.

A BENEFIT

Crazy as it sounds
A benefit of cancer
Is that people tell you that they are glad that you are alive
A fact which sometimes goes unnoticed
Or at least unsaid
For many, oftentimes.

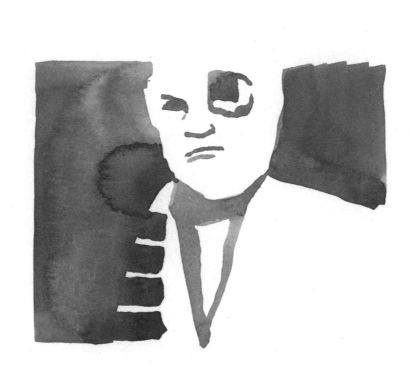

4

RADIATION

*R*adiation, the final leg of my triathlon, was an awful monotony. I showed up Monday through Friday for six weeks, already worn out by eighteen weeks of chemo and a double mastectomy. Every day of radiation I told myself: "Just one more." Reader, I apologize: I don't like to write about it. I was all out of bravery, and I was tired of people calling me Wonder Woman.

Radiation clinics tend to be in the basement because radiation is dangerous and needs to be contained in bunkers, the kind where you hide out during nuclear war. Walking into the clinic felt like walking into a field hospital. The walls were lined with bandaged, bruised, burned people. Beautiful people God made out of his loving heart, hurting and broken.

I'd gathered from websites and other people that radiation was like a sunburn. For most people, I hear it is. It wasn't for me. My skin got pink, and then it hurt, and then it started to blister.

Twenty-four days in, my mom looked at my weeping, sticky skin and said, "You know, honey, I think it would be okay to ask for pain meds." I cried. I cried because it hadn't even occurred to me that it was an option. I thought I just had to be tough. This should be hard, right? They're burning cancer out of me. I showed my chest to a young oncology resident, who immediately gave me a very generous prescription for pain meds.

Twenty-seven days in, three days shy of my thirty treatments, my radiation oncologist looked at my skin—which was hardly there—and said, "Oh." Dismay was written across her face. "That's enough." While stopping the treatment was a relief, it was hard for me to reconcile. Eighteen weeks of chemo, double mastectomy, thirty rounds of radiation. That was always the plan. That was how we were going to kill the cancer. Apparently, I didn't have enough skin for that.

And just like that: nine and a half months of planned treatment were done. Done enough. They bandaged my weeping chest. I walked out the door and drove home, trying to keep my seatbelt from hitting my wounds.

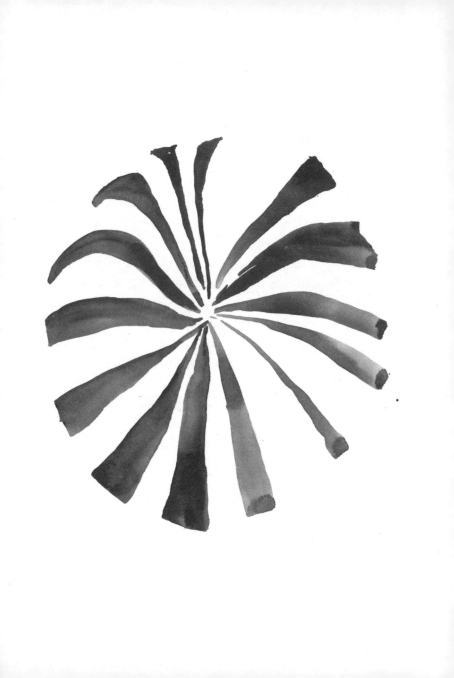

TODAY IS VERY HARD TO DO

Today is very hard to do.
I'd like to wake up in two weeks.
My radiated skin is sore, purple, sticky.
It feels like the organs beneath are, too.
I thought that I was very near a finish line,
Then they moved it—
They just need to take my ovaries,
By the way.
I just can't stop crying.
I can't wait till it's over.

It's dark heavy gray out,
A dirty wet doormat sky.
My skin feels more like an internal organ—
Raw and on the surface.
Despair is not inspiring, not for me.
My palette gets all monochrome
All limited and useless
I feel all limited and useless
Sore knuckles all over my body
Hurting hinges
Swollen swinging doors
Five years where we wonder and then things look pretty good

RADIATION

I hardly wrote during radiation.
Not about radiation, anyway.
About anything but: any distraction.
A daily life-giving death by sandpaper,
Once a day, for 30 days.
So now they are all an amalgam:
Drive to town,
Take the exit,
Right lane, left lane around the parking
Maybe grab coffee at JJ's
Right lane, turn,
Stop sign, turn right into valet parking.
Say hello to Paul, the kind man who takes the car
And knows my name.
(Be kind, you are not the only one hurting.)
In the revolving door, to the right,
Take a breath.
Take the elevator to the basement.
Nurses, EMTs, doctors, people being treated
All bearing God's image, all broken.
(Be kind, you are not the only one hurting,
And you have grace enough to share.)
Down the hall to the waiting room, sign in.

Smile, be kind,
until the day you can't look up anymore or you'll cry.
Be kind when you can't smile, too—
to all of the people around you,
waiting to have something burnt out of them.
Hurting people have the superpower of suffering.
Some won't talk, some won't stop.
Lined up with lasers, I take deep breaths
Listen to the music and motors.
The basilisk stares down my skin with precision
I try to breathe correctly so it hits the right cells,
    wherever they are.
It winks at me, it whines, it bites, it heals.
It goes to sleep, I get dressed, I say thank you to the techs.
Be kind to the techs: they do this all day, every day.
Underground, under fluorescent lights:
They burn hurting people to save their lives.
I am thankful and sorry for them.
I get the hell out of there.

5

THE FINISH LINE MOVED

*C*hemo, mastectomy, radiation. That was the triathlon we had mentally prepared for. Then, Lord willing, we would be done, and just have follow-ups.

I had a professor in music school who told us that a good song was like baseball with two bases: you leave home plate, you go further from home plate, you go back home. Build, tension, release. Completion. That's how you tell a good story. I like that.

Then my oncologist moved the finish line. Nonchalantly. "You could have your ovaries removed." They probably didn't work anymore, anyway. I didn't have to do it, she said, but it would be easier than shots every month to lower my estrogen. I agreed—the fewer days that were tethered to treatment, the better. I wanted to walk further away from cancer and everything associated with it. By the way: I needed to take an estrogen-lowering medicine for five years. Or ten. (We'd arm-wrestle over that later.) That medicine made me feel ninety years old. The bones in my feet made me cry when I stood up in the morning. All of my bones hurt.

People who love me cheered that I was cancer free, and I loved them for it. But while I was grateful, I was too exhausted to celebrate yet. I just wanted to curl up and cry.

Near the end of treatment, my oncologist gave me some advice: "We've been beating you up all year. Be gentle with yourself. Give yourself at least a year to start getting up on your feet." I floated that comment in conversation a lot afterward, as a white flag: Be gentle with me? I am exhausted. I'm alive, hallelujah. I can't wait until I feel like getting out of bed and off the floor. But I am exhausted in every possible way. This feels like a good time to throw in the prophet Jeremiah: "They dress the wound of my people as though it were not serious" (Jeremiah 6:14). Don't do that. They're probably still running their race, and the finish line isn't where they thought it was.

YOU LOVE ME?

*Written and published seventeen years before
cancer, reread a few minutes before my diagnosis.*

You say you love me
I say yes, I know you love me
But I don't really mean it, not as I ought
(and it feels like "ought")
My heart in all its fear and aching
Has emptied the words, dumped out the meaning
And I have put them on my head like a makeshift helmet
To shield me from the shrapnel
Yes, yes, you love me, of course
You're like that, You are faithful and nice and good,
I say
And every word is idolatry, little lessernesses
That I can sort of believe when I hardly believe
Your No smothers my mouth with your kiss
—No to me, made like your lesser lovers.
How dare you water down my wine
When I'm intent on getting you drunk,
Seducing and romancing you
How dare you paint me an impostor,
A dye-cut facade?

You pray to ghosts, you do not cry out to my Spirit
How dare you take these words as a shaming rebuke
When this is the soul-moan of your Lover who longs
To give the fullness of himself
To press his heart into yours
To overwhelm you with his overtures?
I am God made God-man and crossed into frailty and
temptation
I am fully God, fully man, and you are fully Beloved.
Other name calling is all conjecture,
Amateur attempts by those who see as man sees
You are Beloved through and more through
First and now and last
I wooed and won you before you were a twinkle in Adam's eye
Before you drew the breath in your lungs
And right after this
And at 3:36 a.m. when the fallout hits
You have ravished my heart with one look of your eyes.
Treasure, take it for truth.
It courses through you that I am yours and you are mine
And I will come like chemo to kill so you can live
If need be, and it does.

That's my blood I'm chasing it with,
Wine to waken you,
My words are my word
That baffles darkness
And quickens you
And draws you out
And was crushed for the wrongness
That crushes you
That you crush with
Conquers kings
And rescues damsels in dire straits.

AFTER

a few weeks after I finished my treatments, I thought I was having a recurrence. The lymph nodes in my neck were rocks. I dialed the on-call physician in the wee hours of the morning and pulled into the clinic parking lot as the sun came up.

My bloodwork showed that my liver numbers were very high. The young doctor I'd never met was concerned—it might be cancer, metastasized to my liver. I said, "Okay. I hear you. When will you know something? I need to frost cupcakes for my son's birthday party at 4 p.m." No way in hell was cancer stealing this celebration.

In the middle of the party, I got a call that my scans were all clear. Apparently, suddenly taking up intense cross-training right after chemo, surgeries, and radiation can overload your liver. Tire flipping and weights, while empowering, were a bit much. I had lost all sense of listening to my body: I had been tired and in pain for so long that I was numb to signs of stress. My husband and I stepped around the corner from the playground; he held me, and I sobbed.

Cancer steals so much. Time, money, body parts. Energy, hope, happy moments. But it also rips away complacency. Seen against such a dark backdrop, the beautiful parts of life are so good it hurts. I refuse to give cancer credit, to call it a gift. It's a thief, it's anti-life. Something I'd always known as a member of humanity, and had likely spent more time considering than the average American in 2017, suddenly reverberated through me: I am going to die. In a year, in fifty years: I am going to die. But also: *right now*, I am alive. And there are cupcakes.

HOW SHOULD I END
THIS BOOK, WHEN WE ALL
HAVE DIFFERENT ENDINGS?

a book of cancer writing is like a "choose your own ending" book, but you don't get to choose. I don't know if you have cancer, or a friend with cancer. Maybe you have cancer in your rearview mirror; maybe you are years into cancer and know you will have it all of your days, however many they are.

It's hard to tell anyone who's staring at suffering and death that there is hope available at the bottom. Unless you've been down there, maybe you shouldn't. That said, when I am torn up and broken and *do* find hope down here—there—I babble about it. God hovers near to the brokenhearted, to the broken-bodied. Sometimes it's like finding a pack of sparklers and a lighter at the bottom of a well.

Because I've written down these moments, I've met a lot of people with cancer. It's heartbreaking to know so many who have had their hearts and bodies broken in this way. It's wrong, and we know it. And yet: like opals, light can play in the cracks of a broken heart, in spite of the darkness. God comes near to the brokenhearted and holds on tight. He keeps every one of our tears and weeps with us. I can lay my head down, you can lay your head down, on the lover of your soul. And rest.

UP

I can't sleep.
A raucous second line of angels and demons
Race behind my eyes from left to right,
Inklings of thinking run amok.
I turn the light on and write them down.
I sing hymns in my head.
I talk at Jesus out loud.
I pray on paper.
I listen until my ears ring in the silent night.
I lay down, deliriously awake, as the fourth watch begins.
I lay on my left side, sheets over my shoulder.
I try to give up.
Jesus—or was it the third person of the Trinity?
   —comes down.
He lays his hand on me, head to toe.
He pushes me down, gently, into the soft ground of my mind:
"First you have to die
 for me to raise you to life."
I accede and fall under.

ACKNOWLEDGMENTS

I am beyond thankful for the many people who love and encourage me and helped me create something life-giving out of cancer, especially my families and dear friends. Kenny Hutson, I'm so glad we get more years to be together. We know not to take them for granted. Story and Del, I love you so. I'm amazed as God makes you more and more yourselves. Mom and Dad, we really needed you and you were there. Mom, thank you for giving me lots of journals in the backseat of the Volvo. Alice Smith, you've made practically everything I've made better. Tish and Jonathan, the Hutsons love the Warrens.

The first edition of this book was crowdsourced by many, many people. They even provided copies for me to share with my medical and support teams. I've given them to people around the world, to hospital libraries, to palliative care workers and oncologists and nurses and hospices because of your generosity. God bless you. I am so grateful to Jodi Hays for her artwork, and to David King for lending his talents to the independent first edition.

Acknowledgments

Preparing this collection for a second edition, one framed by essays, has been a rich process. Looking at these poems and the years after cancer has been both hard and healing. Good/hard. Thank you to Cindy Bunch and Tianna Haas and all of the IVP team. You all are such good writing midwives. You make me write better, and you make my writing better.